Low Carb Diet

Low Carb Meals and Low Carb Snacks that Satisfy the Whole Family

Linda Stephan

Copyright © 2013 Linda Stephan
All rights reserved.

Table of Contents

TO THE READER 1

CHAPTER 1: RISE AND SHINE WITH A FORTIFIED BREAKFAST 4
    Crunchy Maple Grape Nuts 4
    Healthy Honey Oat Cereal 7
    French Toast Strawberry Dippers 9
    Breakfast Egg Muffins 11
    Cinnamon Raisin Muffins 14
    Asparagus and Mushroom Omelet 16

CHAPTER 2: LUNCHTIME RECIPES FOR AFTERNOON ENERGY 18
    Eggs, Lox and Caramelized Onions on Bagel 18
    Silky Onion Soup 20
    Tuna Salad Supreme in Tortilla Shells 23
    Low-Cal Greek Salad 25
    Spinach Salad with Chicken and Raspberry 27
    Lettuce Roll-Ups with Pumpkin Seed Pate 29

CHAPTER 3: GREAT DINNER SURPRISES 32
    Mushroom Laced Meatballs 32
    Sassy Cheese and Chicken Enchiladas 35
    Colorful Veggie Meatloaf 38
    Grilled Summer Kabobs 40
    Veggie Laced Macaroni and Cheese 42

CHAPTER 4: UNIQUE SIDE DISHES 45
    Fake Mashed Potatoes 45
    Simplistic Green Beans 47
    Dressy Cauliflower Casserole 49

CHAPTER 5: FULFILLMENT WITH DRINKS 51

Pina Colada Smoothie 51
Refreshing Fruit Shake 53
Awesome Juice Spritzer 54
Honey Dew Smoothie 55
Apricot Peach Slush 57
Smooth Strawberry Passion 59
Wean Off of Soft Drinks 61

CHAPTER 6: MAKE AHEAD SNACKS 62
Sweet Popcorn Extravaganza 62
Granola Mini Balls 65
Homemade Sweet Granola Mix 67
Healthy Workout Granola Mix 69
Low-Carb Nachos and Fixings 71
Crispy Fried Fish with Lemon Sauce 73

CHAPTER 7: LET'S HAVE A PICNIC 75
Oriental Cabbage Salad 75
Kickin' Deviled Eggs 77
Chicken Waldorf Salad 79
Fresh Green Bean and Tomato Italiano 81
Confetti Pasta Salad 83
Cobb Salad with Crab 85

CHAPTER 8: EXCITING DESSERTS 86
Chocolate Sponge Cake with Strawberries 86
Luscious Lime Cheesecake Tarts 89
Fruity Bread Pudding 91
Almond Ricotta Pudding 93
Heavenly Chocolate Sorbet 94
Non Traditional Squash Pie 96

CHAPTER 9: WISE WOK COOKING 98
Shrimp Egg Rolls 98
Mandarin Cauliflower and Broccoli Medley 102
Stir Fry Chicken and Peaches 104
Oriental Rice 107
Sweet and Sour Shrimp 109

Pears Cardinal 113

CHAPTER 10: LIST OF LOW-CARB FOODS................ 116

CHAPTER 11: TIPS FOR PREPPING 120

To The Reader

Low calorie diet is a general phrase that can have different meanings. Anyone can eat smaller portions of the same foods they are already consuming, but this doesn't adequately justify a low calorie diet. What you eat makes a huge difference in getting the most out of any type of diet. Advertising trends can misrepresent the true meaning of a low calorie diet, while staying within certain truthful perimeters. This book is designed to bring focus on true low calorie diets, that introduce you to a new way of life. Being stronger, healthier and having more energy, is the goal of a successful low calorie diet.

There will be misconceptions addressed, as you read through the chapters. Facts about preservatives, sugar, grains and drinks, will awaken your thoughts about what you are feeding yourself, and your family. The truth is, a low calorie diet is not just for losing weight, but learning how all foods have a direct affect on your body. Just as you know that cigarettes and large amounts of alcohol are harmful, habits of eating certain foods can weaken you immune system, slow down metabolism, and cause fatty tissue to form in your arteries and veins.

You will also find delicious recipes that are just right for stepping into your new life. If you wish to shed a few pounds, mix and match the recipes and portions, according to the carbs. With each recipe made from low-carb foods, and under 500 calories each, the choices are huge.

Why Calorie Counting is a Lie

Keeping calories low should not involve taking out a book and writing down every calorie of food you eat. That gets real boring, real fast. You simply need to know what types of foods can easily be burned off and which ones, cannot. One of the highest forms of calories that is difficult to unload, is sugar. Look at any label and you will see this word.

According to the American Heart Association, no more than 100 calories of sugar should make up a grown woman's diet in one day. This amounts to 6 teaspoons. For a man, 150 calories, or 9 teaspoons, should be the limit. One bowl of whole-grain cereal with milk, contains as much as 9 teaspoons of sugar.

While this may seem downhearted, it gets even worse. Preservatives play a very important role in adding empty calories and high carbs. Take, for example, a box of macaroni and cheese. You may feel that you are being frugal in selecting a product that has cheese, grain, and vitamins, not to mention a shelf life of a year, but here is the ugly truth. Preservatives contain corn syrup, hydrogenated oil, nitrates or sulfates. While consumption of these ingredients can give you a sensation of fullness, they are very difficult for the digestive system to process. Feeling sluggish, developing heart burn and producing fat, are three real symptoms of consuming processed foods. While the package calories may read, 400 calories per serving, is doesn't tell you that these calories are close to impossible to burn off.

You can make it a habit of counting calories, but unless you start with foods that are good for your body, consuming a low carb diet, will be in vein.

Chapter 1: Rise and Shine with a Fortified Breakfast

Crunchy Maple Grape Nuts

Description

Breakfast should contain energy-packed foods to jump start your day. However, in the hustle and bustle of preparing for the day, many people grab a box of cereal. Instead of breaking this habit, keep your own homemade varieties on hand. Low calorie and delicious, these recipes will give your family the right mix of vitamins in a low carb diet. Make ahead and store in airtight containers.

Yields: 12 Servings

Ingredients

3 cups whole wheat flour
1/2 cup barley flour
1/3 cup oat flour
1/3 cup toasted wheat germ
1/2 cup brown sugar

1/2 teaspoon salt
2 teaspoons baking soda
2 teaspoons maple flavoring
1/4 cup heated honey or maple syrup
1/2 cup low-fat milk
2 teaspoons cinnamon

Instructions

1. Warm oven to 325 degrees.

2. Sift and blend dry ingredients

3. In a separate bowl, beat the liquid ingredients together.

4. Stir liquid ingredients into dry ingredients.

5. If the mixture is too watery, work in additional flour.

6, Spread on 2 or 3 baking sheets and bake for 10-15 minutes. After baking, allow to cool, then break up any large clumps and return to oven for an additional 10 minutes.

7. Cool and store in air-tight container.

Healthy Honey Oat Cereal

Description

Here is another version of homemade cereal for those that love to wake up their mouths with lots of crunch and flavor. Nuts, raisins and sweet natural ingredients make this breakfast cereal a great kick start to the day.

Yields: 12 Servings

Ingredients

4 1/2 cups rolled oats
6 Tablespoons sunflower seeds
12 Tablespoons sliced almonds
6 Tablespoons chopped pecans
6 Tablespoons raisins
6 Tablespoons honey
1/4 teaspoon cinnamon
1/4 teaspoon maple extract

Instructions

1. Warm oven to 325 degrees.

2. Place a small pan over a larger pan of boiling water and add the honey, cinnamon and extract. Heat just until well mixed.

3. Spread baking sheet with aluminum foil and combine all other ingredients (except raisins). You may want to use a baking pan that has a slight lip around the sides, or raise up the edges of the foil to keep dry ingredients from falling off.

4. Using your hands, or a large wooden spoon, mix well, the dry ingredients.

5. Add the honey mixture and coat as much of the dry ingredients as you can.

6. Spread the mixture evenly over the pan and bake for 15 minutes.

7. Remove from oven and let cool. Do not worry if your cereal does not appear crunchy. This comes once it has cooled.

9. After cooling, mix in the raisins and store in an airtight container.

French Toast Strawberry Dippers

Description

Getting kids to the breakfast table is a tough chore. Usually running late, they will grab a finger food, like a doughnut or other gluten-filled treat. Have these quick dippers ready to reach for as they hit the door, and know that they are getting good taste and healthy energy.

Yields: 4 Servings

Ingredients

- 8 slices low-carb sandwich white bread
- 4 Tablespoons softened cream cheese
- 6 fresh, sliced strawberries
- 3 large eggs
- 1/4 cup low-fat milk
- 1 Tablespoon butter
- 1/2 cup maple syrup
- 1/4 cup no-sugar strawberry jam

Instructions

1. Spread cream cheese on 4 slices of bread.

2. Line the cream cheese topping with the sliced strawberries.

3. Top with a bread slice to make a sandwich.

4. In a bowl, mix together the eggs and milk.

5. Use 1/2 of the butter to lightly grease a griddle or skillet and heat on medium.

6. Dip the sandwiches into the egg batter, one at a time, and place in the warmed griddle or skillet.

7. Cook the bread on each side until golden brown. Add remaining butter, if needed.

8. Remove each sandwich, pat with paper towels and cut into 4 long sections.

9. Combine the syrup and jam and heat in a microwave for 30 seconds.

10. Remove and stir well.

11. Place the tasty toast sections in a bread basket, beside the dip, and watch them disappear.

Breakfast Egg Muffins

Description

Use the weekend to cook up a filling and healthy egg breakfast for the day ahead. It will soon become a tradition of a starting a free day, just right, with plenty to go around.

Yields: 8 Servings

Ingredients

8 eggs
½ cup Swiss or Cheddar cheese
½ cup milk
¼ cup chopped onion
¼ cup chopped mushrooms
¼ cup green pepper
¼ cup chopped tomatoes
2 Tablespoons butter
4 plain bagels
8 stale pieces of bread

Instructions

1. Lay out the pieces of bread and cut out the middle in the shape of a circle. This will serve as a pattern for cooking your egg mixture.

2. In a bowl, whisk the eggs and milk together.

3. Blend in the onion, mushrooms, green pepper and tomatoes.

4. Melt 1 Tablespoon butter in a large skillet and arrange the bread patterns.

5. Pour the egg mixture in the center of each bread pattern, lower heat and cover.

6. After about 4 minutes, remove the cover and sprinkle each round egg with cheese.

7. Add extra butter if needed to keep the bottoms from sticking.

7. Turn off heat and recover skillet.

8. Toast ½ bagel and place on a plate.

9. Carefully remove each egg and peel away the outer bread.

10. Place the round egg on top of the bagel, discarding the bread.

Serve with fresh fruit or a glass of juice.

Cinnamon Raisin Muffins

Description

Nothing can compare to fresh, homemade muffins, right from the oven. These treats will satisfy your craving for bread and sweets, but actually give you less than 150 calories each. Vary the ingredients and have a different selection of muffins each week.

Yields: 12 Servings

Ingredients

1 ½ cups flour
1 ½ teaspoons baking powder
½ teaspoon baking soda
¼ cup butter, refrigerated
1 egg
¼ cup sour cream
¼ cup milk
¼ cup raisins
2 Tablespoons sugar, or sugar substitute
1 teaspoon cinnamon

Instructions

1. Heat oven to 400 degrees F.

2. Combine flour, baking powder and baking soda in large bowl.

3. Cut in the butter until coarse crumbs form.

4. Make a well in the center.

5. In a small bowl, beat the egg, then add the sour cream, milk, raisins, sugar and cinnamon, blending thoroughly.

6. Pour the egg mixture in the center of the flour and mix well.

7. Take a muffin pan and either line with paper muffin holders, or grease lightly.

8. Fill each cup 2/3 full.

9. Bake for 15 minutes, or until browned.

Apple butter or fruit preserves can be used to spread on each muffin.

Asparagus and Mushroom Omelet

Description

This dish makes a meaty and tasty meal for not only breakfast, but lunch, as well. With only 5 grams of carbohydrates and 21 grams of protein, per serving, you will pick up extra energy and not get hungry through the course of the day.

Yields: 4 Servings

Ingredients

8 eggs
8 Tablespoons water
12 stalks fresh asparagus
1 cup sliced mushrooms
1 cup low-fat mozzarella cheese

Instructions

1. In a large skillet, add an inch of water and bring to a boil.

2. Add the asparagus, in two or three different sections,

and cook uncovered, just until tender-crisp. Remove and pat dry.

3. Using a large bowl, whisk the eggs and water.

4. Prepare a large skillet by melting 1 Tablespoon butter .

5. When butter reaches a sizzle over medium-high heat, add ½ of the egg mixture.

6. Cook until the bottom of the egg mixture sets.

7. Carefully lift up the edges with a spatula and allow the uncooked portion to flow out and cook.

8. Once the top is cooked thoroughly, add the asparagus, mushrooms and cheese, and fold into a sandwich with part of the egg.

9. Remove the omelet and cut in half. Repeat with the rest of the egg mixture.

Chapter 2: Lunchtime Recipes for Afternoon Energy

Eggs, Lox and Caramelized Onions on Bagel

Description

Afternoons do not have to be a battle with fatigue and a sluggish feeling. Allow your mid-day meal to recharge your body with fulfilling foods that bring nutrition to your organs and pep up your blood flow. You'll never miss the calories, but you will enjoy missing that afternoon slump that used to slow you down.

Yields: 4 Servings

Ingredients

4 teaspoons butter
1 sliced onion
8 eggs
2 Tablespoons heavy cream
4 ounces lox
4 toasted buns

Instructions

1. Melt 2 teaspoons butter in a skillet, add sliced onions, and cook over medium heat for 8-10 minutes, or until golden brown. Remove to a plate.

2. Beat eggs and cream in a bowl.

3. Melt remaining butter in the skillet and add mixture from bowl.

4. Add salt and pepper, to flavor, and stir constantly, until almost set.

5. Add lox and onions, stirring until heated throughout.

6. Spread on toasted bagel halves.

Silky Onion Soup

Description

Enjoy this tasty soup with a few carrot sticks and a piece of Melba toast. The creamy rich flavor will remind you of an elegant evening meal, instead of a lunch time treat.

Yields: 8 Servings

Ingredients

3 Tablespoons butter
1 sliced onion
2 garlic cloves, minced
2 leeks (white part only), cut in 1/2" strips
1 medium zucchini, sliced
½ teaspoon tarragon
¼ teaspoon salt
¼ teaspoon pepper
2 cups scallions, thinly sliced
28 ounces chicken broth
1 ½ cup water
½ cup heavy cream

Instructions

1. Melt 2 Tablespoons butter in a saucepan, over medium heat.

2. Add onion, garlic, leeks, zucchini, tarragon, salt and pepper.

3. Cover and simmer about 7 minutes
4. Stir in 1 ¾ cup scallions and cook until wilted.

5. Add broth and water and increase the heat until all is boiling.

6. Reduce heat and simmer for 10 minutes.

7. Remove from heat and break up the vegetables with a masher.

8. Return to a medium heat and add the remaining butter and the cream.

9. Heat just until boiling begins.

10. Remove from heat and sprinkle with remaining scallions.

Makes a great make ahead meal for warming up when

on the run.

Tuna Salad Supreme in Tortilla Shells

Description

Give new meaning to tired tuna salad that grows old after a time or two. The right mix of veggies and a complementary bowl will turn tuna into a sought after lunch.

Yields: 4 Servings

Ingredients

4 8-inch round flour tortillas
1 Tablespoon olive oil
3 5-ounce cans Albacore tuna, drained
6 stalks celery, chopped
1 cucumber, peeled and cubed
2/3 cup mayonnaise
16 cherry tomatoes, quartered
4 lettuce leaves

Instructions

1. Heat oven to 400-degrees.

2. Take 4 oven-proof bowls and turn upside down.

3. Brush both sides of the tortillas with olive oil and place one over each bowl.

4. Bake in the oven until the tortillas are crisp and hold their shape, about 7 to 10 minutes.

5. Remove from oven and keep draped over the bowls until completely cooled.

6. In a bowl, mix the remaining ingredients (except the lettuce leaves).

7. Invert the bowls and lace each one with a lettuce leaf before adding the tuna salad.

You will never eat tuna salad on bread again!

Low-Cal Greek Salad

Description

Never miss out on the taste of feta cheese, blended perfectly in a luscious bed of romaine lettuce. Here is a great way to give in to your taste bud desires, without adding unwanted carbohydrates.

Yields: 1 Serving

Ingredients

8 leaves romaine lettuce, torn
1 cucumber, peeled and sliced
1 chopped tomato
½ cup red onion, sliced
½ cup low-fat feta cheese, crumbled
2 Tablespoons olive oil
2 Tablespoons fresh lemon juice
1 teaspoon dried oregano leaves
½ teaspoon salt

Instructions

1. Mix torn lettuce, cucumber, tomato, onion, and

cheese in a large serving bowl.

2. Using a separate bowl, whisk together the oil, lemon juice, oregano, and salt.

3. Pour over salad.

Spinach Salad with Chicken and Raspberry

Description

Raspberry adds a tangy flavor to salads and chicken, so why not combine them? Adding a few other tricks will make this mid-day meal something to look forward to.

Yields: 4 Servings

Ingredients

¼ cup white vinegar
5 Tablespoons olive oil
1 teaspoon honey
½ teaspoon orange peel, shredded
½ teaspoon salt
¼ teaspoon pepper
4 skinless, boneless chicken breast halves
5 cups torn spinach
5 cups torn mixed greens
1 cup fresh raspberries
1 papaya, peeled, seeded and cubed

Instructions

1. Combine the vinegar, 4 Tablespoons olive oil, honey, orange peel, salt and pepper.

2. Pour into an airtight jar and shake well. Store in the refrigerator to chill.

3. In a large skillet, heat over medium heat and add the remaining oil .

4. Add the chicken breasts and cook for 10 to 15 minutes, turning often, to brown all sides.

5. When no longer pink, remove from the skillet and pat out any excess oil and water.

6. Cut the warm chicken into thin strips.

7. In a large bowl, toss the greens, spinach and chicken strips.

8. Take your salad dressing and pour over the salad, tossing well.

9. Add the raspberries and cubed papaya, tossing gently.

Lettuce Roll-Ups with Pumpkin Seed Pate

Description

Move over hamburgers. This flavorful rendition of what used to be a sandwich, will make you wonder why anyone would choose meat over fresh veggies. Filled with marinated vegetables and seasoned with a unique pate, all your friends will want your recipe.

Yields: 6 Servings

Ingredients

6 large lettuce leaves

Marinated Vegetables:

2 stalks celery, sliced in 2-inch strips
1 cup carrots, shredded
¼ cup red onion, thinly sliced
2 Tablespoons flax oil
2 teaspoons lemon juice

Pate:

1 ½ garlic cloves
juice from 1 squeezed lemon
1 cup pumpkin seeds, soaked and sprouted
¼ cup flax oil
¾ teaspoon salt
¼ cup fresh parsley
¼ cup fresh basil
¼ cup dill
1/8 teaspoon turmeric
½ teaspoon fresh rosemary

Instructions for Pate

1. Using a food processor, place the garlic and pumpkins seeds inside and chop.

2. Add the lemon juice and mix until creamy.

3. Add the herbs and seasonings.

4. Pulse to finely chop all the herbs.

5. Spoon into a bowl.

Instructions for Assembly

1. Place all ingredients for marinated vegetables in a

medium bowl and coat all pieces.

2. Lay flat a lettuce leaf and spread on a generous amount of pate.

3. Add ½ cup of marinated vegetables.

4. Roll up, folding the top and bottom to secure.

Chapter 3: Great Dinner Surprises

Mushroom Laced Meatballs

Description

You don't have to tell the family that they are on a low calorie diet when serving up dishes that are guaranteed to hit the spot. Lean hamburger will be anything, but boring, when dressed up with the right spices. See if anyone believes you when you admit that this dish has only 300 calories per serving.

Yields: 6 Servings

Ingredients

1 pound ground beef
1 egg
1/2 cup whole wheat bread crumbs
4 ounces shredded cheddar cheese
1/4 cup onion, chopped
1 Tablespoon Worcestershire sauce
1 Tablespoon fresh parsley, chopped

1/2 teaspoon basil
1/2 teaspoon pepper
1 Tablespoon oil
1 cup sliced mushrooms
1/2 cup beef broth
1/2 cup cooking wine

Instructions

1. Mix together meat, egg, bread crumbs, cheese, onion, Worcestershire sauce, parsley, basil and pepper.

2. Shape into 12 meatballs.

3. Add oil to skillet and brown meatballs on all sides, about 5 minutes.

4. Remove meatballs and dry on paper towels.

5. Add mushrooms to the drippings in the skillet and cook over medium heat for 2 to 3 minutes.

6. In a small bowl, mix flour, broth and wine until blended.

7. Pour over mushrooms and cook until boiling, stirring constantly.

8. Turn down heat and simmer sauce for 2 minutes.

9. Add meatballs to the creamy mixture and warm thoroughly, before serving.

Sassy Cheese and Chicken Enchiladas

Description

Kids will come running when they smell the succulent aroma of one of their favorite meals. Chicken enchiladas always top the favorites list, especially when dripping with cheese sauce. Microwave the entire meal and save time.

Yields: 6 Servings

Ingredients

2 cups cooked chicken breasts, chopped
1/2 cup chopped onion
1 garlic clove, minced
1 Tablespoon oil
4 ounces chopped green chilies
1/2 cup chicken broth
2 teaspoons chili powder
1 teaspoon cumin
4 ounces cubed cream cheese
6 6-inch flour tortillas
1/4 pound Colby or Cheddar cheese, cubed
2 Tablespoons milk

1/2 cup fresh chopped tomato

Instructions

1. In a 2-quart microwavable dish, mix onion, garlic and oil.

2. Microwave on high for 2 minutes. Stir and return for 1 more minute.

3. Remove and add chicken, chilies, broth and seasonings. Blend well.

4. Return to microwave and cook on high for 4 minutes.

5. Remove and add cream cheese, stirring until all the cheese is melted.

6. Spoon 1/2 cup of the mixture onto a tortilla shell and roll up. Repeat 6 times and place all, seam side down, on a flat microwavable dish.

7. In a clean microwavable dish, mix the Colby or Cheddar cheese, milk and 1/4 cup tomato and microwave on high for 1 minute. Stir and return for another 1 or 2 minutes.

8. Remove the cheese sauce and pour over the enchiladas.

9. Microwave on high for 4 minutes.

10. Remove and top with remaining tomatoes.

11. Return to the microwave and cook on high for another 2 to 3 minutes.

Serve with salsa and chips.

Colorful Veggie Meatloaf

Description

Put sparkle in an old dish by using creative, and healthy vegetables. This one dish meal will add new meaning to meatloaf, as it was once known.

Yields: 8 Servings

Ingredients

1 1/2 pounds lean ground beef
3 cups white bread crumbs, toasted
1 cup diced tomatoes
1 cup fresh or frozen green beans (thawed)
1 egg
1 carrot
2 Tablespoons Worcestershire sauce
1 1/2 teaspoons salt
1/4 teaspoon pepper
1/4 cup ketchup

Instructions

1. Preheat oven to 375 degrees F

2. In a large bowl, mix all ingredients (except ketchup), until well blended.

3. Turn into a loaf pan and top with ketchup.

4. Bake for 50 to 60 minutes, or until cooked throughout.

5. Remove and transfer to a platter, patting dry any excess fat.

Serve with a tossed salad for a filling, low calorie dinner.

Grilled Summer Kabobs

Description

Grilling during the spring and summer months can be exciting. The smell of meat that is char-broiled to perfection, can get your tummy growling. Make a delightful and low carb dinner, while including steak. A little bit goes a long way with this recipe.

Yields: 6 Servings

Ingredients

1 1/2 pounds boneless beef sirloin steak, cut into strips
1 zucchini, cut in 1-inch pieces
1 squash, cut into diagonal pieces
2 onions, quartered
12 cherry tomatoes
1/2 cup mayonnaise
1/2 cup plain yogurt
1/4 cup lemon juice
3 cloves garlic, minced
2 teaspoons minced ginger root
1/2 teaspoon cardamom
1/2 teaspoon cumin

1/2 teaspoon coriander

1/8 teaspoon red pepper

Instructions

1. Prepare the marinade by blending all seasonings, mayonnaise, yogurt and lemon juice. Put 1/2 cup of dressing aside for later.

2. Skewer the steak strips between the zucchini, squash, onions, and tomatoes.

3. Place the kabobs on a hot grill and brush with the marinade.

4. Grill for 10 or 15 minutes, or until the meat reaches the required doneness, turning and brushing twice.

5. Remove and serve with the reserved dressing.

Veggie Laced Macaroni and Cheese

Description

Macaroni and Cheese, from a box, offers little in the way of low carbs and vitamins. However, it will not take long for family to miss this simple mix of cheese and pasta. Try this homemade version that has a new twist and watch them ask for more.

Yields: 4 Servings

Ingredients

9 ounces penne noodles
1 ½ cups sharp cheddar cheese
1 Tablespoon tarragon
1/8 teaspoon ground white pepper
4 carrots, peeled and sliced
juice from one fresh orange
¼ cup water

Instructions

Warm oven to 350 degrees F.

In a saucepan, combine the carrots and juice from orange.

Add 1/4 cup water and heat until boiling.

Turn down, cover and simmer for about 30 minutes.

Remove from heat and transfer to a blender.

Puree contents.

In a separate pan, boil the penne noodles in salted water until al dente.

Drain off the water, reserving 1 cup in the pan.

Add the drained pasta to the pan, along with the puree.

Heat on medium, stirring to coat penne.

Cook, stirring often,
Add 1 cup cheese, tarragon and white pepper.

Once the mixture becomes creamy, pour all into a greased baking dish.

Add the remaining cheese on top and bake for 20

minutes.

Remove and let stand for 5 minutes before serving.

Chapter 4: Unique Side Dishes

Fake Mashed Potatoes

Description

If your family craves meat and potatoes, this is just an old habit. However, you can give them what they want by serving a meat dish and using this unique recipe for mashed potatoes, made from fresh cauliflower. The flavor will be better, the consistency, fluffy, and that mindset of meat and potatoes will quickly dissipate.

Yields: 4 Servings

Ingredients

1 fresh cauliflower head
1 Tablespoon water
1 Tablespoon butter
2 Tablespoons heavy cream

Instructions

Chop cauliflower into small pieces and add to a large

casserole dish.

Add 1 Tablespoon water, cover, and microwave on high for 5 minutes.

Remove and let stand for 5 minute.

Drain water from cauliflower and place in a food processor.

Add butter and heavy cream.

Process until smooth.

Scoop out and place in a serving bowl.

Simplistic Green Beans

Description

Sometimes the best things in life are amazingly simple. Take this green bean dish, for example. Only two ingredients deliver taste and fulfillment, complimenting any main dish.

Yields: 4 Servings

Ingredients

1 pound fresh green beans
1 onion, cut in half and sliced thick
1 Tablespoon oil
2 Tablespoons butter
Unrefined sea salt and pepper to taste

Instructions

Using a heavy skillet, sauté green beans, over medium heat, in oil and 1 Tablespoon of butter.

Add onion pieces and continue sautéing until the onions brown.

Turn into a serving bowl and let guests season, to their liking, with salt and pepper.

Dressy Cauliflower Casserole

Description

Cauliflower is a great food for keeping carbs low, but can become quite boring when prepared over and over again. This recipe dresses up this vegetable by using other seasonings for a flavor that almost makes you forget about the main ingredient.

Yields: 6 Servings

Ingredients

1 fresh head cauliflower, broken up, or 1 16 ounce frozen bag, cooked and drained
½ cup onion, diced
1 ½ cup fresh mushrooms
2 Tablespoons butter
¼ cup heavy cream
¼ cup mayonnaise
4 ounces shredded cheddar cheese
¼ cup green onions, chopped

Instructions

Warm oven to 350 degrees F.

Place prepared cauliflower in a greased 2-quart casserole dish.

In a skillet, sauté onion and mushrooms in the butter.

Add to the cauliflower and mix.

Mix in cheese.

In a small bowl, combine cream and mayonnaise.

Pour the sauce over the cauliflower mix and coat well.

Sprinkle the top with green onions.

Bake, covered, for 25 minutes.

Remove lid and bake another 10 minutes, or until the top is brown and crispy.

Chapter 5: Fulfillment with Drinks

Pina Colada Smoothie

Description

Soft drinks and some fruit drinks can be loaded with sugar. By side-stepping this calorie boosting substance, drinks take on a more lasting flavor, keep you from tiring and give your body the liquids that they need.

Yields: 2 Servings

Ingredients

1/2 cup unsweetened coconut milk
1/4 cup plain yogurt
1/2 cup fresh pineapple chunks
1/4 teaspoon coconut extract
1 teaspoon fresh lime juice
8 ice cubes
2 packets sugar substitute
2 lime slices

Instructions

1. In a blender, add all ingredients (except lime slices).

2. Blend on high until smooth.

Add a slice of lime to the edge of each glass to add a zesty twist.

Refreshing Fruit Shake

Description

Shakes do not have to weigh you down with unhealthy calories and leaving you feel sluggish. Try this homemade version of a strawberry milkshake and forget the tired feeling. Double the recipe to share with a friend.

Yields: 1 Serving

Ingredients

1 cup strawberries
1 cup almond flavored low-fat milk
1 packet sugar substitute
1 cube tofu
1 cup ice cubes

Instructions

1. Blend together strawberries, milk, sugar substitute, and tofu in a blender.

2. Add ice cubes and blend again.

Awesome Juice Spritzer

Description

Keeping the kids (and adults) away from soft drinks can be a never ending chore. Keep a 2-liter bottle of refreshing juice spritzer in the frig and no one will even miss the pop.

Yields: 6 Servings

Ingredients

9 ounces pineapple, orange, or pomegranate juice
48 ounces club soda or sparkling water

Instructions

1. Add juice to club soda or sparkling water, using a 2 liter air tight bottle.

Freshly processed and strained fruit can also be used in the place of juice.

Honey Dew Smoothie

Description

Add variety to your beverages by using a little thought of ingredient. The flavor will bring a new twist to boring fruit juices. Light and healthy, this drink only has 110 calories per serving. Increase ingredients to share with family and friends.

Yields: 2 Servings

Ingredients

4 cups cubed honey dew
2 apples, peeled, cored and cubed
2 kiwi fruits, peeled and sliced
3 packets sugar substitute
2 Tablespoons lemon juice
2 cups ice cubes

Instructions

1. Combine all ingredients (except ice cubes) in a blender and blend well.

2. Add ice cubes and blend until ice becomes broken into small pieces.

Apricot Peach Slush

Description

This fruity drink has become a favorite of diabetics because of the sweet flavor and smooth texture. It's hard to think that something so refreshing can be good for you, but it is. Keep plenty of apricot nectar on hand because this beverage will go fast.

Yields: 6 Servings

Ingredients

15 ½ ounces apricot nectar, chilled
2 fresh peaches, peeled, pitted and sliced
1 ½ cups crushed ice
1 Tablespoon lemon juice
1 ½ cups chilled carbonated water

Instructions

1. In a blender, combine the apricot nectar, peaches, lemon juice and crushed ice.

2. Blend until smooth.

3. Spoon into a tall glass, filling halfway.

4. Fill the glass to the top with carbonated water.

Smooth Strawberry Passion

Description

Forget the milkshakes and all the calories and instead, make up a batch of Smooth Strawberry Passion drinks. Low in carbs and fat, this drink is great for a gathering or just to sit on the porch on a hot summer day.

Yields: 6 Servings

Ingredients

4 cups fresh strawberries, sliced
1 banana
1 kiwi fruit
16 ounces vanilla yogurt
1 cup ice cubes

Instructions

Using a blender, add strawberries, banana, and yogurt.

Blend until creamy.

Add ice cubes, one at a time, blending until they are

broken up.

Pour in glasses, garnishing with kiwi fruit.

Wean Off of Soft Drinks

In a world of perfection, you would cut out all soda. The sugary sweeteners, found in soda, is almost impossible to break down. However, the addiction to soft drinks can cause you to abandon a new eating plan, after a day or two. If you currently have sugary soda in your daily life, definitely change to a diet brand - but don't try to cut it out cold turkey. You want to succeed in your new diet, so it is okay to start out slow. Slowly wean yourself off of the addictive, artificial taste by trading for a more refreshing taste of natural ingredients.

Chapter 6: Make Ahead Snacks

Sweet Popcorn Extravaganza

Description

Showtime in front of the TV will become even more exciting when there is a big bowl of crunchy, sweet snacks ready for each turn. Make this light and wholesome finger food ahead of time and keep in an air tight container.

Yields: 8 Servings

Ingredients

4 Tablespoons butter, melted
2 egg whites
2 packets sugar substitute
½ teaspoon vanilla extract
½ teaspoon cinnamon
¼ teaspoon salt
1 ½ cups low-carb cereal flakes
3 ounces pecans or almonds
4 cups pop corn

Instructions

1. Heat oven to 300 degrees F.

2. Lay a sheet of aluminum foil over a baking sheet and spray with Canola oil.

3. In a small bowl, combine butter, egg whites, sugar substitute, vanilla, cinnamon and salt.

4. Whisk the egg mixture until well blended.

5. Using a large bowl, add cereal and nuts and coat with the melted butter.

6. Add popcorn and lightly toss.

7. Pour mixture onto the baking sheet and spread evenly.

8. Bake for 20 to 25 minutes, or until crispy.

9. Remove and cool.

Store in an air tight container until show time. By adding the popcorn to the mixture last, there will be less clumps for hands to grab.

Granola Mini Balls

Description

These little bundles are the perfect size for snacking or grabbing as a quick energy picker-upper. Leave a plateful on the table and the refrigerator door will have less activity.

Yields: 6 Servings

Ingredients

2 cups granola
½ cup raisins
½ cup pecans, chopped
½ cup dried apricots
1 cup low-fat dried milk
1 cup creamy peanut butter
1/3 cup honey

Instructions

1. In a large bowl, mix granola, raisins, pecans, apricots, dried milk, and honey.

2. Gradually add peanut butter, stirring until all ingredients are well covered.

3. Using your hands, form into small balls and place on small squares of waxed paper.

4. Place the balls, including the waxed paper on a serving plate. The waxed paper will keep the balls from sticking to one another.

Homemade Sweet Granola Mix

Description

Teach your kids how to have a great snack by letting them help make this sweet, crunchy treat. They will learn how to eat healthier, plus have something to munch on while playing video games.

Yields: 8 Servings

Ingredients

1 cup rolled oats
1 cup almonds
1 cup unsalted peanuts
1 cup raw sunflower seeds
1 cup flax seeds
1 cup sweetened coconut flakes
1 cup dried cranberries
3 Tablespoons brown sugar syrup

Instructions

1. Preheat oven to 250 degrees F.

2. Line a baking sheet with parchment sheets.

3. Use a large mixing bowl and add all ingredients.

4. Mix well with a wooden spoon or spatula.

5. Spread onto the baking sheet and flatten.

6. Bake for 15 minutes.

7. Remove and break up the granola pieces.

8. Bake for an additional 15 minutes.

9. Remove and cool.

10. Place into an airtight container.

Healthy Workout Granola Mix

Description

Here is another type of granola treat that is favored by athletes after a good workout. However, it was soon found to be a favorite of youngsters, as well.

Yields: 8 servings

Ingredients

1 cup rolled oats
1 cup almonds
1 cup dried cranberries
1 ½ cups butter
½ cup brown sugar
2 Tablespoons honey
½ teaspoon vanilla extract

Instructions

1. Preheat oven to 375 degrees F.

2. Coat baking tray with spray canola oil
3. In a large bowl, combine the oats, almonds, dried

cranberries, and ground cinnamon.

4. Blend well with a large wooden spoon or spatula.

5. Add the butter, brown sugar, honey and vanilla extract together in a separate bowl, blending well.

6. Pour the butter mixture into the dry ingredients and mix until all is coated.

7. Spread the mixture onto the greased baking tray and press down to flatten.

8. Place in the oven for 20 to 25 minutes.

9. Remove and cool.

10. Either cut into bars, or break up the pieces for a bite size treat.

Low-Carb Nachos and Fixings

Description

Many people admit that their toughest part of staying on a low-carb diet, is giving up chips. Here is a unique way to have it all. Chips, cheese, salsa, at an amazing 6.5 net carbs. The secret is in the chips and here is a way to have your cake and eat it, too.

Yields: 10 Servings

Ingredients

8 ounces low-carb soy chips
1 cup chopped black olives
4 ½ ounces chopped, mild green chilies
12 ounces cheddar cheese, grated
2/3 cup sour cream
2/3 cup salsa

Instructions

1. Move rack in oven to within 6 inches of the broiler and preheat to broil.

2. Line 2 baking sheets with aluminum foil and spray lightly, with canola oil spray.

3. Arrange the soy chips on the baking sheets in a single layer.

4. Top each chip with olives and chilies.

5. Sprinkle with cheese.

6. Place in oven and broil for 45 to 60 seconds.

7. Remove and transfer to a platter.

8. Place sour cream in one small bowl and the salsa in another.

9. Serve together.

Crispy Fried Fish with Lemon Sauce

Description

Who says you can't have fried fish on a low-carb diet? Choose pollock, whiting, haddock or scrod, and don't forget the sauce.

Yields: 4 Servings

Ingredients

4 8-ounce fish fillets
1 egg
2 ounces baked potato chips, ground
2 Tablespoons water
2 Tablespoons canola oil
½ cup mayonnaise
3 Tablespoons fresh dill, chopped
2 teaspoons lemon zest, grated
¼ teaspoon pepper

Instructions

1. Spread chip crumbs on a flat surface lined with waxed paper.

2. In a wide bowl, whisk 1 egg with water and brush on each fillet.

3. Heat a non-stick skillet to medium heat and add 1 Tablespoon canola oil
4. Dredge each fillet through the crumbs and place in the hot skillet.

5. Turn each fillet once after cooking about 3 to 4 minutes, or until golden brown.

6. Gently remove to plates
7. In a small bowl, mix the mayonnaise, dill, zest and pepper for dip.

Chapter 7: Let's Have a Picnic

Oriental Cabbage Salad

Description

Summer comes with lots of potlucks and bar-b-ques. Trying to watch your eating habits can be very trying with hamburgers and hot dogs being served. Start bringing great side dishes to get togethers and introduce the crowd to great tasting foods.

Yields: 4 Servings

Ingredients

½ head grated, green cabbage
3 chopped scallions
2 Tablespoons sesame oil
2 Tablespoons rice wine vinegar
2 Tablespoons toasted sesame seeds

Instructions

1. In a large serving bowl, combine the cabbage,

scallions, oil and vinegar.

2. Toss well, then refrigerate.

3. Right before serving, add the sesame seeds and toss lightly.

Kickin' Deviled Eggs

Description

Deviled eggs are an all time favorite at picnics, but these beauties will make the crowd stop and say, WOW! The special ingredient may surprise you, and certainly, anyone who indulges. With 1 gram of carbs and 178 calories, maybe it won't hurt to have a couple.

Yields: 20 eggs

Ingredients

10 large eggs
4 Tablespoons cream cheese
½ cup mayonnaise
2 Tablespoons fresh chives, minced
2 teaspoons wasabi paste
pepper
1 teaspoon sea salt

Instructions

1. Boil eggs in a single layer, using a large saucepan, for 7 minutes.

2. Turn off heat and cover saucepan for 15 minutes.

3. Drain water off and refill with cold water. Let stand for at least 10 minutes.

4. Peel eggs and cut in half, long way.

5. Remove yolks and place in a large bowl.

6. Add the cream cheese and wasabi paste.

7. Mash with a fork or masher until everything is blended and resembles small crumbs.

8. Stir in the mayonnaise and chives and add pepper to taste.

9. Place the yolk mixture in a pastry bag and squeeze filling into the white cups of the eggs.

10. Make a swirling motion, beginning with the outer layer and working to a point in the middle.

11. Just before serving, sprinkle with sea salt.

Chicken Waldorf Salad

Description

Everyone loves the flavor of apples and walnuts, mixed with greens and a tart dressing. Make it a meal by adding chicken and using a new kind of dressing that will make guests request, time and time again.

Yields: 4 Servings

Ingredients

4 cooked and cubed chicken breasts
1 cup chopped celery
1 ½ cup chopped apples
4 ounces walnut pieces
4 Tablespoons raisins
1 cup low-fat Italian dressing
10 cups Iceberg and Bibb lettuce

Instructions

1. Place the lettuce, chicken, apples and celery in a large serving bowl and toss well.

2. Pour the Italian dressing over all and toss to coat.

3. Add the walnut pieces and raisins, gently blending.

Fresh Green Bean and Tomato Italiano

Description

There is nothing more flavorful than the taste of fresh green beans that are served up steamed and crunchy. Bring this dish to your outdoor party and you will find that even the youngsters will be temped with their presence. This is a quick and easy side dish that delivers a compliment to any type of meat.

Yields: 6 Servings

Ingredients

3 cups fresh green beans
2 plum tomatoes, sliced into thin wedges
2 Tablespoons fresh basil
¼ cup Italian dressing

Instructions

1. Steam green beans for 10 minutes, just long enough to remove the raw texture.

2. Cool and add tomatoes and basil.

3. Pour dressing over all and toss lightly, just to coat.

Confetti Pasta Salad

Description

Here is a dish that is almost too beautiful to eat. Colorful and robust, it will seem more like a main dish than a complimentary side. Increase the size to share for an outdoor BBQ or other picnic event.

Yields: 4 Servings

Ingredients

1 cup multicolored, low-carb penne, cooked
4 artichoke hearts, diced
4 ounces thinly sliced turkey breast strips
8 ounces fresh mozzarella, diced
4 Tablespoon red pepper
8 Tablespoons fresh, chopped green beans
4 Tablespoons olive oil
4 teaspoons balsamic vinegar
2 teaspoons fresh oregano, chopped

Instructions

1. Combine pasta, artichoke hearts, turkey, mozzarella,

red pepper and green beans in a large salad bowl.

2. In a small bowl, mix oil, vinegar, and oregano.

3. Pour over the pasta mixture and toss.

Cobb Salad with Crab

Description

Seafood is the main ingredient that gives this salad a wonderful flavor. Along with other cobb salad favorite additions, this side dish goes very well with those lake-caught fish.

Yields: 4 Servings

Ingredients

12 cups romaine lettuce, torn into bite-size pieces
12 ounce cooked crab meat
2 cups cherry tomatoes, halved
1 cup crumbled blue cheese
½ cup olive oil raspberry flavored dressing

Instructions

1. In a large serving bowl, add lettuce, crab meat, tomatoes and blue cheese.

2. Toss well then add dressing and toss again.

Chapter 8: Exciting Desserts

Chocolate Sponge Cake with Strawberries

Description

There is something wrong with a low-carb diet that does not allow for the sweet pleasures in life, mainly cake and chocolate. This dessert will satisfy both with rich flavor and texture.

Yields: 10 Servings

Ingredients

7 egg whites
1/8 tsp cream of tartar
¾ cup sugar
3 egg yolks
1 teaspoon vanilla
1 cup cake flour
3 Tablespoons melted butter
1 ½ ounces semisweet chocolate
2 Tablespoons canola oil
12 plump strawberries

Instructions

1. Heat oven to 350 degr F.

2. Use a large bowl to beat the egg whites and cream of tartar until foamy.

3. Add the sugar, gradually, while whipping into a meringue, with soft peaks.

4. In another bowl, beat together the egg yolks and vanilla.

5. Add the egg yolk mixture to the egg whites, gradually, folding until well blended.

6. Fold in the flour, stirring until all has been absorbed.

7. Pour batter into the cake batter and fold gently.

9. Spoon the batter into a 10-inch tube pan and bake for 35-40 minutes, or until the center proves clean, with a tooth pick.

10. Remove the cake and turn upside down on a large bottle so all sides are exposed to the air.

11. Cool for about an hour.

12. Remove the pan and run a knife along the sides of the pan to loosen the cake, then invert onto a wire rack to further cool.

13. Place on a serving dish.

14. Melt the chocolate and oil, slowly to keep from scorching and drizzle over the cooled cake.

15. Dot the top with strawberries.

Luscious Lime Cheesecake Tarts

Description

Cheesecake can add the final touch to a great meal, or be a special treat for friends that visit. Adding the tartness of lime and the sweetness of kiwi, will let you savor every bite.

Yields: 12 Servings

Ingredients

12 vanilla wafers
¾ cup cottage cheese
8 ounces low-fat cream cheese
¼ cup sugar or sugar substitute
2 eggs
1 Tablespoon grated lime rind
1 Tablespoon fresh lime juice
1 teaspoon vanilla
¼ cup vanilla flavored yogurt
2 kiwis, peeled, sliced and halved

Instructions

1. Using a 12-cup muffin pan, line each cup with a paper muffin liner.

2. Heat oven to 350 degrees F.

3. Place a vanilla wafer in the bottom of each cup.

4. Using a blender, add the cottage cheese, cream cheese and sugar. Blend well.

5. Add the eggs, lime rind, lime juice and vanilla. Beat until smooth.

6. Spoon the mixture into the lined muffin cups and bake for 15-20 minutes, or until well set.

7. Remove from oven and chill completely.

8. Right before serving, spread the vanilla flavored yogurt on top and garnish with kiwi pieces.

Fruity Bread Pudding

Description

Bread pudding can become a sinful dish when laced with peaches and cream. Serve up this delightful dessert to family and friends. Have the recipe ready to share because everyone will want to know your secret ingredients.

Yields: 12 Servings

Ingredients

1 teaspoon butter, softened
6 slices low-carb bread, cubed
1 ½ cups fresh or frozen chopped peaches
4 eggs
1 cup heavy cream
½ cup sugar
¼ teaspoon nutmeg
1 ½ teaspoons vanilla
2 Tablespoons sliced almonds

Instructions

1. Warm oven to 350 F degrees.

2. Butter an 8-inch square baking dish

3. Add bread crumbs and peaches to dish and toss.

4. In a medium-sized bowl, add eggs, cream, sugar, nutmeg and vanilla, and whisk together.

5. Pour the egg mixture over the bread and peaches.

6. Let stand for 10 minutes to allow the bread to absorb the liquid mixture.

7. Sprinkle almonds on top of the dish.

8. Place the dish inside a 9x11 pan, filled with boiling water. The water should rise halfway up the sides of the 8-inch dish.

9. Bake for 45 to 50 minutes, or until a clean knife shows that it is done.

Almond Ricotta Pudding

Description

Take a break with a smooth, luscious pudding that is satisfying and only 8 carbs per serving. Quick to make, this recipe is designed for 1 serving but can be stretched to include the whole family.

Yields: 1 Serving

Ingredients

½ cup ricotta cheese
¼ teaspoon almond extract
1 packet sweetener
1 teaspoon slivered toasted almonds

Instructions

1. Mix the ricotta cheese, almond extract and sugar substitute.

2. Sprinkle with almonds.

Enjoy.

Heavenly Chocolate Sorbet

Description

Remember the fudge ice pops that you enjoyed as a child? Here is an adult version that will bring back memories, yet satisfy the grown up you. You will need an ice-cream maker for this recipe. This treat is not for kids, the more reason to sneak away and enjoy.

Yields: 4 Servings

Ingredients

2 cups ice cold water
1 teaspoon unflavored gelatin
1 ½ cups sugar-free chocolate syrup
1 cup low-fat milk
3 Tablespoons dark rum

Instructions

1. Add 2 Tablespoons ice water in a glass measuring cup.

2. Sprinkle with gelatin.

3. Microwave for 20 seconds to dissolve the gelatin.

3. In a medium-sized bowl, add ¾ cup syrup, the remaining ice water, milk and rum.

4. Stir until blended.

5. Add the remaining chocolate syrup into the mix and whisk.

6. Add the dissolved gelatin and stir.

7. Pour the mixture into an ice-cream maker and churn, according to instructions.

8. Remove and place in an airtight container and place in the freezer until ready to serve.

Non Traditional Squash Pie

Description

Pumpkin pie may be the tradition, but there's a new version in town. Serve up this wonderful dessert that offers much lower calories and carbs and start a new traditional during the holidays, or any time.

Yields: 8 Servings

Ingredients

3 cups cooked winter squash, mashed
¾ cup unsweetened coconut milk
¼ cup honey
3 eggs
2 teaspoons pumpkin pie spice
1 ½ teaspoons maple extract
1 ½ Tablespoons arrowroot powder
1 ¼ teaspoons unrefined sea salt, finely ground
½ teaspoon sugar

Instructions

1. Warm oven to 350 degr F.

2. Mix all ingredients with a mixer or in a food processor. If the consistency is too thick, add a little water, 1 teaspoon each, until no longer stiff.

3. Pour into a greased 10-inch pie pan and bake for 50 to 60 minutes, or until a knife comes out clean, when placed in the center.

4. Allow pie to cool then chill for another 30 minutes, to firm.

Chapter 9: Wise Wok Cooking

Shrimp Egg Rolls

Description

Reintroduce your wok to keep fat and sugar limited. It may take some time to prepare these awesome egg rolls, but the results are well worth the trouble.

Yields: 8 Servings

Ingredients

½ pounds raw shrimp, cleaned and deveined
1 teaspoon sherry
1 teaspoon salt
½ teaspoon cornstarch
3 Tablespoons canola oil
3 cups diced celery
½ teaspoon sugar
1 Tablespoon water
½ cup fresh bean sprouts
1 cup shredded lettuce
1 cup chopped water chestnuts

16 egg-roll wrappers

Instructions

1. In a small bowl, combine shrimp, sherry, salt and cornstarch.

2. Let the mixture marinate for 12 to minutes.

3. Heat 1 tablespoon oil in work.

4. Add shrimp mixture and stir-fry until shrimp is pink and firm.

5. Remove to a mixing bowl.

6. Add remaining oil to wok and add celery, stir-frying for 2 to 3 minutes.

7. Add sugar and water.

8. Cover and let steam for 1 minute.

9. Remove cover and stir-fry until all the liquid has evaporated.

10. Add to shrimp mixture.

11. Add remaining ingredients.

12. Blend well.

13. Prepare wrappers by laying out flat.

14. Fill each one with ¼ cup shrimp mixture.

15. Lift lower triangle of wrapper over filling and tuck the point under.

16. Leave the upper point of the wrapper flat.

17. Bring the 2 end flaps up and over the enclosed filling and press flaps down firmly.

18. Brush cold water over the exposed triangles and roll the filled portion until you have a neat package. The water will seal your ingredients protectively.

19. Repeat until you have 16 filled egg rolls.

20. Fill the wok with 3 inches of oil in the center.

21. Heat to 375 degrees F.

22. Using tongs, lower 4 eggs rolls into the oil and deep fry for 3 to 4 minutes, or until golden brown.

23. Drain on paper towels, blotting out all of the oil.

24. Repeat until all egg rolls have been cooked.

Serve with hot mustard, plum sauce or soy sauce. You can also store for later use by cooling and wrapping in plastic wrap, then placing in freezer bags to refrigerate or freeze.

Mandarin Cauliflower and Broccoli Medley

Description

Making your vegetables more interesting, will create a reason for your family to try any new variation. The aroma of this mixture, while stir-frying, will have everyone sitting at the table, ready to enjoy.

Yields: 4 Servings

Ingredients

2 Tablespoons canola oil
½ teaspoon salt
10 mushrooms, sliced lengthwise
1 small onion, minced
1 cup water
1 ½ cups bite-size cauliflower pieces
1 ½ cups bite-size broccoli pieces
½ cup water
2 teaspoons sugar
2 teaspoons cornstarch dissolved in 1 Tablespoon water

Instructions

1. Heat oil and salt in wok.

2. Add mushrooms and onion.

3. Stir-fry for 2 minutes or until tender.

4. Add water and bring to a boil.

5. Cover and steam for 5 minutes.

6. Uncover and add broccoli.

7. Cover and steam for an additional 10 minutes, stirring occasionally.

8. Uncover and add remaining water and sugar.

9. Bring to a simmer and add cornstarch mix.

10. Stir until sauce thickens and all vegetables are well coated.

Stir Fry Chicken and Peaches

Description

A delicate sauce make this stir fry chicken recipe a hit with the family. Low-cal and nutritious, peaches all extra flavor to a classic sweet and sour classic dish.

Yields: 6 to 8 Servings

Ingredients

1 3-pound chicken, cut into 8 pieces
1 teaspoon salt
½ teaspoon poultry seasoning
3 Tablespoons cornstarch
1 cup canola oil plus 1 Tablespoon oil
1 clove garlic, peeled and crushed
8 ounces frozen sliced, unsweetened peaches, thawed
1 Tablespoon sugar
2 Tablespoons lemon juice
½ cup chicken broth
2 teaspoons cornstarch dissolved in 1 Tablespoon water
10 ounces frozen snow peas
3 cups hot cooked rice

Instructions

1. Fill wok half full with water.

2. Place chicken pieces in a shallow baking dish and sprinkle with salt and poultry seasoning.

3. Place dish on a wire rack atop the wok and cover.

4. Cover chicken and turn wok on medium-high.

5. Steam the chicken for 45 minutes.

6. Remove and dry chicken pieces.

7. Rub cornstarch into each chicken piece.

8. Remove water from wok and wipe dry.

9. Add 1 cup canola oil into wok and heat to just under sizzling.

10. Fry chicken pieces in the hot oil, 2 or 3 pieces at a time until lightly browned.

11. Remove to a plate, lined with paper towels.

12. Pour oil out of wok and discard.

13. Add 1 Tablespoon oil to wok, add garlic, and stir-fry until brown.

14. Remove and discard garlic.

15. Add peaches and sugar, snow peas, stirring into the garlic liquid.

16. Stir in lemon juice.

17. Add chicken broth and heat to boiling.

18. Stir in dissolved cornstarch.

19. Add snow peas, stirring into the liquid.

20. Cover and steam for 30 seconds.

21. Add chicken pieces to wok and cover.

22. Steam for 30 seconds or until chicken is heated.

Serve over hot cooked rice.

Oriental Rice

Description

It seems that every time you have a Chinese-type of meal, there is tons of white rice left over. Put it to good use with this tasty oriental rice recipe. It will make a great side dish for a lunch or dinner menu
Yields: 4 to 6 Serving

Ingredients

1 Tablespoon oil
2 cups cold cooked rice
½ cup chopped water chestnuts
½ cup raisins
¼ cup soy sauce

Instructions

1. Heat oil in wok.

2. Add rice and cook, stirring until coated with oil.

3. Add water chestnuts and raisins.

4. Stir-fry until all is heated.

5. Add soy sauce and blend well.

6. Turn into a serving bowl.

Small portions of left over meat can also be used for additional flavor.

Sweet and Sour Shrimp

Description

Who doesn't love the awesome flavor of sweet and sour sauce, mixed with shrimp and fresh vegetables. Here is a recipe that will amaze your taste buds and satisfy your hunger.

Yields: 4 Servings

Ingredients

1 carrot, peeled and diagonally sliced
1 green pepper, cut into 1-inch squares
2 cups canola oil
½ teaspoon salt
8 ounces breaded, frozen shrimp
1 clove garlic, peeled and flattened
1 cup unsweetened pineapple chunks, drained (save the juice)
¾ cup mixed sweet pickles, drained

Sauce Ingredients

1 ¼ cup unsweetened pineapple juice

¼ cup white wine vinegar
1 Tablespoon soy sauce
1/3 cup brown sugar
1/4 cup catsup
2 Tablespoons cornstarch

Instructions

Prepare the Sweet and Sour Sauce first.

1. In a small saucepan, combine 1 cup pineapple juice, vinegar, soy sauce, sugar and catsup.

2. Stir over medium heat until simmering.

3. Dissolve cornstarch in ¼ cup pineapple juice and add to pan.

4. Stir until smooth.

5. Remove from heat and set aside.

Stir-Fry Section
1. Place carrot slices in saucepan and cover with water.

2. Boil for 5 minutes
3. Add green pepper and boil for another 5 minutes.

4. Drain and set aside.

5. Add oil and salt to wok.

6. Heat to 375 degrees F.

7. Fry the frozen shrimp, a few at a time, until lightly browned.

8. Drain on paper towels.

9. Remove oil from wok and wipe clean with paper towels.

10. Discard oil.

11. Add 1 Tablespoon oil to wok.

12. Set to high heat.

13. Add garlic, rubbing against sides and bottom until lightly browned.

14. Remove and discard.

15. Add peppers and carrots.

16. Stir-fry for 30 seconds.

17. Add the sweet and sour sauce.

18. Next, add the pineapple chunks and pickles.

19. Stir-fry until hot.

20. Add cooked shrimp and cover all with sauce.

21. Spoon over hot cooked rice.

Pears Cardinal

Description

No one will find these pears boring with the succulent flavor of raspberries, surrounding them. Easy to make while you have your wok out, or use your stove top. Attractive, rich and melt-in-your mouth consistency, make this dessert a great finish to any meal.

Yields: 8 to 10 Servings

Ingredients

6 ripe pears
Red food coloring
20 ounces frozen raspberries, thawed (or fresh is even better)
2 Tablespoons sugar
2 teaspoons cornstarch, dissolved in 2 Tablespoons water
¼ cup kirsch liqueur, or raspberry flavored syrup

Instructions

1. Place a rack in wok that is filled with simmering water.

2. Stand up pears on the rack and cover.

3. Steam for 10 to 15 minutes.

4. Remove pears from rack.

5. Run under cold water to gently remove skin.

6. Rub each pear with a little red food coloring for a blushed appearance.

7. Refrigerate until chilled.

8. Blend raspberries in a blender.

9. Strain out seeds.

10. Place the raspberry puree in a saucepan and bring to a boil.

11. Stir in sugar and dissolved cornstarch.

12. Keep stirring until mixture thickens.

13. Remove from heat and add liqueur or flavored syrup.

14. Refrigerate until well chilled.

15. When ready to serve, place on pear in a serving dish and spoon the sauce over the top.

Chapter 10: List of Low-Carb Foods

Trying to keep all of the terms straight, like carbohydrates, calories, low-fat, and induction, can be difficult to understand. Not all low-carb foods are low-fat, or low in calories. Start with this list of foods that can keep anyone on the straight and narrow in beginning a low-carb diet. After awhile, you will learn, just by tasting, how some foods dull your palate in enjoying the rich flavor of natural foods. One of these is sugar. It is a known fact that refined sugar decreases your ability to savor flavor. By ridding your diet of refined sugar, bleached white flour, margarine, and other processed, synthetic additives, you will begin to enjoy the wholesome flavor that low-carb natural foods have to offer.

- Cucumbers
- Broccoli
- Iceberg Lettuce
- Celery
- White Mushrooms
- Turnips
- Radishes
- Romaine Lettuce

- Asparagus
- Green Pepper
- Okra
- Cauliflower
- Cabbage
- Red Bell Pepper
- Spinach
- Beets
- Green Beans
- Carrots
- Kale
- Sugar Snap Peas
- Corn
- Onions
- Watermelon
- Strawberries
- Cantaloupe
- Avocado
- Blackberries
- Honeydew Melon
- Grapefruit
- Oranges
- Peaches
- Papaya
- Cranberries
- Plums
- Raspberries
- Pineapple
- Nectarine
- Blueberries

- Apples
- Pears
- Kiwi Fruit
- Cherries
- Tangerines
- Mango

If you feel that you just can't stay away from refined sugar, try these natural alternatives in cooking and see how quickly your habit begins to fade.

- Molasses
- Sorghum
- Real Maple Syrup
- Maple Sugar
- Sucanat or Rapadura
- Agave Syrup
- Coconut Sugar
- Honey

Bread is a real obstacle for many that have grown up on products made from white flour. If you are able to find bread products with any of the following main ingredients, you will be doing your body a favor.

- Corn
- Soybeans
- Oat Bran
- Barley

- Organic Sprouted Wheat
- Millet

Pasta has grown popular in making quick meals but the ingredients can be full of carbs. While many companies are slow to transform a popular-selling product into one that offers good nutrition, one company is gaining ground because of the low-carb content. Known as Shirataki, the starch is made from the root of devil's tongue, a type of yam. While you will probably never find this product in your local grocery store, keep your eyes open for new types of pasta alternatives in the foreign cuisine section.

Chapter 11: Tips for Prepping

People raised in countries, outside of the United States, are constantly amazed at how our grocery shopping is done. They are used to shopping for fresh produce and seafood on a daily basis, not weekly, as is practiced in the states. How can anything be fresh when it is allowed to set for a week?

To say that it is simple to eat healthier on a low carb diet, according to American standards, would be misleading. Manufacturers of ready-made food stuffs , count on the fact that there is too little time to spend on healthy eating. Popping a cardboard box into the microwave or opening a can, has replaced wholesome foods with convenience. Unfortunately, this way of thinking has led us to where we are today. Weight gain, inadequate vitamin supply, and slow metabolism, is the result of pumping your body with preservatives and sugars that prevent a healthy system. While time is on everyone's mind, there are some short cuts that you can take to prepare for low carb meals.

Freeze, Freeze, Freeze

In the summer, fresh vegetables are everywhere. But

when winter sets in, finding produce can make your search for fresh foods, a real chore. This year, snap up those great looking veggies and freeze so you will have plenty on hand during the winter months.

Not all vegetables freeze well. Those with a high water content can become mushy and less flavorful, like onions and cucumbers. But many other types can retain their shape, presence and vitamins, for meal prepping. Here are some examples of vegetables that can be frozen and ready to use:

- Asparagus
- Beans
- Broccoli
- Cauliflower
- Squash and Zucchini
- Eggplant
- Snow Peas

How to Properly Freeze:

It is not difficult to prepare vegetables for future use, but it does take a little bit of planning. Pick a day for putting up your family's favorite veggies and follow these simple instructions to make an ample supply.

Supplies needed:

- 3-quart Saucepan
- Wire Basket
- Jelly roll pan
- Waxed paper
- Freezer Bags
- Marking Pen

Instructions for Blanching

Select your veggies and prepare by cleaning, cutting and making meal ready.

Fill the saucepan half full of water and bring to a boil.

Put the prepared veggies into the wire basket and plunge into the boiling water for 3 minutes.

Remove and drain. Pat dry to remove any excess water.

Line the jelly roll pan with waxed paper and lay out your vegetables in single file.

Place the jelly roll pan in the freezer, just long enough for the food to freeze.

Remove and place in freezer bags, squeezing out as much excess water, as possible.

Mark and date each bag and return to the freezer.

By getting into the habit of preparing garden fresh vegetables for future use, you can rest assured that your family will receive no preservatives or additives from packaged foods.

10 Tips for Staying on a Low-Cal Plan

No one claims that it is easy to break bad habits, but if you look at where you are, and where you want to be, anything is possible. Remember when you thought that using a cell phone was the most impossible thing you had ever done? But now you probably wonder how you ever lived without it. Everyone dislikes change but when the future turns out for the better, you wonder how you ever thought differently. Try some of these tips and you will soon be forgetting about those bad eating habits.

1. Use coconut as a sweetener. Why is coconut downplayed so much? It is a wonderful, sweet and tasty type of low-carb accessory that can become irreplaceable. Use it in main dish recipes, savor the juice and discover that it is very addicting.

2. Who started the rumor that eggs were bad? Eggs are

a great source of protein and can be eaten alone or used in salads and meals. They are also very portable for a quick energy boost. Use to make sauces, to add texture to foods, or just as a snack in the middle of the day.

3. Never throw leftovers away. You just spent a lot of time on a low-cal meal for your family and believe it or not, you have some scraps to deal with. You already know how goo they are for you so wrap them up and use on a salad for lunch tomorrow.

4. Herbs are better than salt. We all have the habit of salting everything that is set in front of us. Break this habit by keeping a variety of herbs close by. The selection will be interesting and fun, plus a lot better than salt, which does nothing but harm your body.

5. Rice is a great filler but not the best when it comes to nutrition. Try something different, like ground cauliflower. The taste will not be so ho-hum and you might just trick your brain into thinking that it is rice, but somehow, even better.

6. Make good use of your muffin pan. Part of the problem with staying on a low- carb diet menu, is thinking that you are going to starve. The portions seem so tiny and your mind just cannot grab hold of the fact

that you will ever be satisfied. Start using a muffin pan to fill with portions so you will get used to having enough. Start with something filling, like pudding or chicken salad. You will be surprised just how much a muffin cup can hold.

7. Salads can be the spice of life. How many other foods are so flexible to accept fruit, meat, and vegetables, without ruining the taste? In addition, dressings and sauces can be an endless supply of flavor. From cheeses to herbs, lemons and limes, you can transform a salad into any flavor you desire.

8. Think of a lettuce leaf as a piece of bread and the need to be fulfilled with a sandwich, will slowly fade away. Wraps are becoming popular with anything and everything. Meat, cheese, pickles, or a mixture of favorite foods. Iceberg lettuce has big meaty leaves for wrapping up tuna salad, eggs, chicken breast, and more.

9. Go on an adventure to an Asian store and look at the labels of pasta. You will probably see some words that are foreign to you, but more than likely, they represent roots and vegetables instead of chemical additives that you do recognize. Asians are not big on bread and grains that make them feel sluggish. Ask someone in the market about the ingredients, or write down the names

and search for yourself.

10. If sweets are your downfall, don't deprive yourself and make the craving worse. Enjoy some chocolate or puddings that can be found on a low carb diet food list. Make ahead to keep on hand for when that craving hits.

Deciding to go on a low-carb diet is not just a choice for losing weight, but changing the way that you look at food. Our society has become accustomed to eating anything that announces 'low-fat' or 'low-carb, that we have been brainwashed into accepting almost anything. Always shop for fresh, or frozen, and learn to enjoy the taste of food that has been replaced with high fat and glucose filled preservatives. Not only will you feel better, but your weight will automatically begin to burn off and give you more energy.

Lightning Source UK Ltd.
Milton Keynes UK
UKHW021446260321
381037UK00008B/2115